HOW I HELP MY PATIENTS LOSE UP TO 30% OF THEIR WEIGHT

EVIDENCE BASED MEDICAL WEIGHT LOSS THAT IS HIGHLY EFFECTIVE

MARTYN CHILVERS M.D.

ISBN: 9798657523140

Printed in the United States of America

This book is dedicated to my two daughters,
Lisa & Candice Chilvers who have inspired me. Without
their support this book would not have been written.

"Many of life's failures are people who did not realize
how close they were to success when they gave up."
Thomas A. Edison

Table of Contents

Introduction

Hello. I'm Dr. Martyn Chilvers, Medical Director of the Triad Weight Loss Clinic in Sarnia, Ontario, Canada. Thank you for your interest in learning how to lose up to 30% of your current weight by following my methodology. After 32 years of practicing as a family physician I retired and for the last 5 years, I have developed my interest and practice in weight management. As a family doctor I never really knew how to help my patients who suffered from obesity yet I saw them suffering. Many of them suffered physically, emotionally, and socially as a result of their weight trouble. I was all too familiar with the medical consequences of obesity and felt I'd like to help these folks more and this led to my development of a medical weight loss clinic and the writing of this book. In the past, the orthodox medical system has largely neglected the management of obesity mainly because we did not have the tools, nor knowledge to correctly manage this medical condition. Fortunately, this is changing. Reading this book and following the advice herein will guide you on the path to successful permanent weight loss. I do suggest reading from the beginning to the end so that all concepts are understood in a logical order.

I'd also like to make it clear that the opinions expressed in this book are my own although they are derived from the teachings from some of Canada's leading weight-loss experts.
I have not been paid by anyone to promote any medication or treatment regimen.

CHAPTER 1

Obesity Bias & Expectations

Thank you for your interest in learning how to lose up to 30% of your current weight by following my methodology.

Okay, so the initial topic is on Obesity Bias. It's important that I address this first because it helps you understand the issues that are interfering with your successful weight loss. Unfortunately, Obesity Bias and the misunderstanding of the overweight is incredibly prevalent in our society today. And it greatly interferes with the management of weight loss. This bias and the stigma associated with obesity is seen all around us – in our government, in our health insurance industry, in our health system and indeed, in society as a whole including you the person who is suffering from weight trouble.

The bias arises at least in part because of societies belief, that obesity is under a persons' control and that the obese person could be thin if they wanted to or chose to. Society feels that the obese person could be thin if only they tried harder, exercised more and ate healthily. I'm here to tell you that this is absolutely not true. Being obese is not a choice. Being obese is not your fault. These beliefs of society though are also ingrained in many of you who are obese. Because of a misunderstanding of what causes obesity patients are often reluctant to take weight loss medication. Medication by some is seen as a crutch rather than a tool. You likely believe that you should be able to lose weight on your own or you remind yourself that you have achieved weight loss before so you should be able to do it again. This time you promise you will keep it off for good. You as well falsely believe that you should be able to control your food intake and lower your weight through sheer willpower. You might feel that you should not have to rely on medication to assist with your weight loss. Other patients accept that they need medication to help them lower their weight but believe that once they are at their target weight, they then should be able to maintain their weight themselves by embracing a healthy lifestyle. These beliefs are a manifestation of obesity bias.

Unfortunately, those who are obese are suffering from a neuroendocrine disorder, a medical condition that prevents them from maintaining their target weight and this medical condition requires lifelong treatment. Would you feel that you don't need medication to control your blood pressure? Or that once your blood pressure is controlled, that you no longer need the medication, as you should be able to control your blood pressure yourself? Probably not.

We realize that we have no direct control over our blood pressure – and so we should realize that we have no direct control over our weight. This is an example of a weight bias that I frequently see in obese patients. As a society, we have come to believe that obesity is a choice – a chosen lifestyle, even. We have even come to believe the stereotypes of overweight and obese people as being somewhat more slow, lazy and gluttonous. All of this is of course totally incorrect nonsense.

As you will learn in this series, obesity is very often a consequence of your genetics along with environmental factors that are largely beyond your control. Obesity is a chronic disease that comes about through no fault of your own – it's a manifestation of a mismatching of brain evolution when food was scarce with our current environment when food is plentiful.

I mention brain evolution because it's largely our brain that determines our food intake. Obesity is a consequence of the neurohormonal drives that evolved in times of food scarcity. Think about it! We used to have to go out and hunt and gather food to survive, and strong mechanisms have developed to ensure our survival. But today, your groceries, your ready-made and cooked meals can be delivered to your door with no more effort than typing a few keystrokes on your phone.

Obesity has become the last area where discrimination is still acceptable within our society, although this is beginning to change. It's just not acceptable to weight-discriminate, and body-shaming or obesity-stigmatizing need to be seen for what they are – examples of shameful behaviour. I found that many of my obese patients have low self-esteem and a sense of inadequacy and even despair. They blame themselves. "I'm too weak-willed!" they'll say. "I've tried before and I've never really succeeded, I'm a major failure at this." Or "I don't like exercise and I am no good at sports." These thoughts that you somehow lack the necessary character traits to lose weight make you feel bad about yourself and can further interfere with your success.

Stop it!

Say to yourself: My obesity is a progressive chronic medical condition. It has occurred through no fault of my own and it requires treatment, just like any other chronic medical condition. Like high blood pressure or diabetes.

You might well be thinking, "But I've tried all the diets and although I've had some short-term success, none of them have worked for me in the long run."

If that's what you're thinking, you are correct: diets don't work. Apart from suggesting a healthy diet like the Mediterranean Diet, your treatment isn't very much about following a specific diet. It's about changing behaviours and taking medication like you would for any other chronic medical condition.

Consider that you have never really had proper treatment for your medical condition. Consider that. Furthermore, consider that you have never had evidence-based medical treatment for your obesity, treatment that has been medically proven to be effective.

You're not a failure. You simply have never had the right treatment before. What I'm trying to accomplish in this chapter is to change the narrative from shame and blame to the narrative of a chronic medical condition that requires treatment. You might ask, "Why does it require treatment? I feel just fine in my own skin. You're still trying to shame me."

My answer is this:

- Obesity is an unhealthy medical state.

- It is associated with at least 40 other medical conditions.

- It puts you at increased risk of developing any one of 11 types of cancer.

Think about it...

We also know that obesity can also lead to:

- social problems

- psychological problems

- financial problems

- shorter life expectancy.

4

We have good medical reasons to treat obesity and the medical model is recently becoming successful.

In the past, doctors really didn't have the right tools to help patients effectively.

A number of patients say to me, "Dr. Chilvers, I already know it's bad for me. But don't bother telling me all the details and statistics. Just tell me what to do."

They don't seem to want to know what obesity can do to the body. Certainly, denial can be useful – in the short term – in minimizing psychological discomfort.

Recall that I've said that obesity is a chronic disease, and like many chronic diseases, it requires self-management by the patient, just like diabetes requires self-management, but under the guidance of a knowledgeable physician. Self-management requires knowledge and education.

Consider this book the start of your education so you have a framework to build your knowledge and skills upon.

Now I'd like to introduce the concept referred to as 'Best Weight', a concept developed by Dr. Freedhoff and Dr. Sharma. You probably are familiar with the concept of ideal weight – that so-called perfect weight for perfect health. For so many patients this so-called ideal weight is simply not achievable, given their specific genetic makeup, whereas we could all strive to achieve our Best Weight.

Your Best Weight is the weight your body naturally stabilizes at while you're living your healthiest lifestyle that you can truly enjoy – and the lowest weight you can sustain over the long term.

My goal is to help you achieve your personal Best Weight. An athletic runner looks to achieving their personal best, even though it may not be the Olympic Best.

Hey – we are not all born to have the physique of Greek gods.

When we humans lose weight, we lose it more rapidly at first and then the rate of weight loss slows as we approach our best weight, and plateaus at this weight. If one uses weight loss medication as well as following a healthy diet, the plateau is lower. And if one combines the medication with cognitive restructuring, your best weight will plateau even lower still.

You might be interested to learn that the reason the rate of weight loss slows is not so much because your metabolism slows, but because you start eating more. Most people don't notice or appreciate that they are eating a little more. The biology of your brain is very powerful on getting you to change your behaviour, in part because on a primitive subconscious level it thinks you are starving to death and it simply won't let you do that!

Losing weight is not natural. So, we are trying to thwart nature and change the natural course of your neurohormonal biology, which is why weight loss is so difficult and such a struggle. This means that it is normal and natural to have difficulty losing weight and to keep it off.

As a doctor, I am always trying to thwart nature and interfere with the natural course of disease.

—

CHAPTER 2

The Role of Diet, Exercise and Calorie Deficit

Diets don't work! That is, they don't work in the long run. Sure, you can follow a diet for a few weeks or even a few months and you can lose weight, but you can't keep it off.

I have mentioned that obesity is a chronic disease, and being a chronic disease, it requires a chronic treatment for the rest of your life. Most if not all diets are restrictive. Diets advise denial, restriction, deprivation and white-knuckle determination. Nobody can keep that up forever.

Typically, diets have varying degrees of short-term success but folks can't maintain their diet long-term, and so this approach fails.

Please don't consider yourself a failure because this approach didn't work for you. It doesn't work for anyone. You're not a failure. Remember – your neurohormonal biology is driving your weight to regain and defending against weight loss. Losing weight is not natural!

So, what should you eat? Well, in order to lose weight, you should take in the least amount of calories that you can still enjoy. So, I'm saying that enjoying food and using it to socialize is part of who we are as humans, and denying yourself is unnatural and unsustainable. Think of your lifestyle as taking in the least amount of calories but still enjoying life. If it feels like deprivation, then you are not enjoying it, and you will not be able to keep it up.

This might look like one piece of chocolate cake instead of two, or it might look like fruit salad instead of chocolate cake, but at the end of the day, you should not feel deprived.

As a doctor, I really want to advocate healthy eating behaviours that tend to

- promote reduced cardiovascular risk

- reduce cancer risk, and

- promote an eating lifestyle that is associated with longevity.

So, in general, I promote the Mediterranean Diet which is associated with better health outcomes. The Mediterranean Diet is not so much a diet as it is a lifestyle of healthy eating. It's a lifestyle that encourages the consumption of all food groups but promotes those that give the most health benefit. The Mediterranean Diet emphasizes plant-based foods namely fruits, vegetables, grains, nuts and seeds. Seafood is consumed at least twice weekly. Cheese and yoghurt at least twice weekly along with moderate proportions of chicken, turkey and eggs on occasion. The consumption of other meats and of sweets are only used occasionally, like once or twice a month. Cooking with herbs and extra virgin olive oil is also promoted. Replace refined grains with whole grains. Choose brown over white. So use whole wheat pasta and whole-grain bread and brown rice instead of white rice.

Because you are cutting back on meat you do need another source of high-quality protein. So, replace meat with a diet high in beans and lentils as these are a good source of high-quality protein from the vegetable kingdom. Beans and lentils or are also a good source of fibre, antioxidants and vitamins.

What I love most about the Mediterranean lifestyle is its focus on social connection through food, as opposed to eating alone. It's all about activity: walking with family & friends, dancing, celebrating and sharing home-cooked food. So when opportunity permits, please eat with family and friends as much as you can and enjoy having a good time while you're eating.

Although I love this Mediterranean diet, from a weight-loss perspective I'm a diet agnostic not recommending any particular diet over the other, but advocate using a diet or eating lifestyle that one can stick with for the long term. If you think you can stick to the Mediterranean Diet long-term, this is the one that I would suggest as being amongst the healthiest.

To be clear, I am not a trained dietician or nutritionist, so I don't involve myself much in dietary counselling with my patients as there are others who are more knowledgeable and trained to counsel in nutrition. I do often refer to Lisa Chilvers, a registered holistic nutritionist who does a wonderful job of working with my patients to perfect a healthy eating lifestyle (Lisa, by the way, happens to be my daughter). Please check out her website at lisachilvers.ca and consider following her healthy eating lifestyle that she refers to as The Loving Kindness Method. It works for her patients. I have had heartwarming feedback from so many of them on what a wonderful job she is doing and how much she has helped them. You might think that a plant-predominant diet is boring and not very tasty, but I can verify personally that this is not correct. Lisa knows how to make this type of healthy eating wonderfully tasty and sustainable in the long term.

Let's move on to the topic of exercise or what I preferred to call activity. Exercise doesn't have to be a formal exercise in the gym or on the track. It can simply be an increase in activity that gets your heart pumping and your lungs breathing harder. If you're like me, when you think of exercise you think of running, and when you think of running, you think of the last time that you ran. Maybe it was a painful and somewhat boring experience. You got out of breath easily and had to stop frequently. No one likes a painful, difficult experience and we all have a normal, natural tendency to avoid pain and unpleasantness. But fortunately, for most of us, walking is not painful and walking is natural.

I do not mean to discourage running if that is your passion, but if you do go down that path, I suggest starting slow, gradually increasing your pace and distance as you get fitter from the training effect. It's easier that way and hence you are more likely to persevere.

I'd now like to list the merits of walking:

1) It assists with weight loss.

2) It improves cardiovascular fitness.

3) It reduces the risk of heart attack and stroke.

4) It improves mental health. It reduces the risk of depression and helps reduces anxiety and
          feeling stressed.

5) It reduces the risk of developing diabetes and certain cancers (colon, breast & uterine).

6) It reduces the risk of developing osteoporosis and associated fracture risk.

7) It may help cognitive function and reduce the risk of developing dementia.

8) It boosts your immune system – which might be useful in these times.

9) It extends your life and

10) Apart from being a solitary exercise, it can be also be enjoyed with family and friends.

I'm going to focus on #1: Assists with weight loss. I advocate walking as an adjunct to weight loss for the reasons above and because it's something that most of us are actually able to do. Running a marathon or training for a pentathlon is not something us mere mortals are able to do. For those of you who are limited by severe arthritis in your knees or hips, cycling or swimming might be substituted. Unfortunately, it takes a fair amount of walking to make a significant impact on your weight. This is why I advocate a daily brisk walk of an hour a day, every day. Even walking can be challenging for a variety of reasons... lack of fitness, poor muscle strength, lack of time, lack of energy, lack of motivation, boredom, cold or rainy weather, etc., etc.

So, start off walking 30 minutes per day every day, and after a few weeks gradually step it up to 1 hour per day every day. This can become a part of your new healthy lifestyle. I recommend walking with a partner if possible, (spouse, neighbour, friend, dog) as chatting as you walk makes the experience more enjoyable. If you do not have a partner, then listening to music or the radio can be enjoyable and help boost energy and reduce boredom.

The weather in Canada is a definite challenge. If it's sub-zero with a vicious cold wind, then dress appropriately. Thermal underwear, thermal gloves, socks and boots and a balaclava with ski goggles will ensure no skin is exposed and help keep you toasty warm!

The walking prescription is challenging, so start off slower and shorter, then gradually increase to the target of a brisk daily walk of an hour. One could certainly break it up into two 30-minute walks if one preferred. Do not sabotage your hard work by rewarding yourself with, say, a small bag of potato chips. 275 calories? Easy come, not so easy to go. Don't let an hour of hard work evaporate in a minute of indulgence.

A few words of caution:

1) If you develop chest distress (pain, tightness) while you are active, you need to stop the activity and seek medical attention before resuming the activity.

2) If we are still social distancing, your walking partner cannot be someone who doesn't live with you.

Now, when you lose weight you are not necessarily just losing fat. You are at risk of losing muscle as well which is undesirable for several reasons. This includes the loss of muscle which ends up lowering your resting metabolic rate and this, in turn, makes it more difficult for you to keep the weight off. Now walking does help to reduce loss of muscle in the biggest muscle groups in your body i.e. your legs and buttocks so this actually is an additional benefit of walking. Adding weight training to your activity will greatly reduce the loss of muscle associated with weight loss and help you to tone up your muscles. Apparently, it doesn't take a lot of weight training to accomplish this. Simply exercise your major muscle groups twice a week using heavy weights where your muscles fatigue after 12 repetitions. So those light girly weights that you ladies have aren't going to cut it.

Now to be clear, activity in the form of exercise, in general, is not an easy or efficient way to lose weight, but following the active lifestyle may contribute to about 10% of your weight loss, so increasing your activity helps you derive all of the health benefits and contributes to your weight loss.

In short – try to burn as many calories as you can while still enjoying a healthy lifestyle. If you find it's a chore, though, you won't do it for long. This is human nature. This is normal. Try to find an activity that you enjoy and can keep up for the long term.

Also, remember: physical activity alone results in very modest weight loss benefit, and so it must be paired with dietary intervention to achieve optimal weight reduction. You cannot walk off an unhealthy diet. Studies have shown us that patients who are successful in keeping the weight off also keep up an active lifestyle long-term.

I would now like to review with you the concept of a caloric deficit. To lose weight you have to have a caloric deficit. That is, you have to burn more calories than you consume.

To give you an idea: there are about 3500 calories in 1 lb. of fat. If you develop a caloric deficit of 500 calories per day, this would add up to 3500 calories per week, which would enable you to lose 1 lb. of fat per week. One way of ensuring that you will have a caloric deficit is to consume no more calories than your resting basal metabolic rate.

You can calculate your basal metabolic rate by using an online calculator. Now because your basal metabolic rate goes down as you lose weight, I'd suggest recalculating it with every 20 lbs of weight loss. I'm also an advocate of tracking calories and to maintain caloric tracking for a year or so.

There are many popular apps that you can download on your smartphone that make it very easy to track your caloric intake. MyFitnessPal is probably the most popular tracking mobile app although I personally use YAZIO to track my intake. We know from clinical studies that patients who track their caloric intake and track their activity tend to be more successful overall so there is good reason to be bothered to track calories and activity.

After a year, tracking closely may not be necessary, as the habits you've developed have hopefully become ingrained. It is educational and illuminating to track your calories, and you'll be surprised when you learn that there aren't as many calories in foods you thought were high in calories, and vice versa. You can also make it fun by becoming a "calorie detective", discovering where all the calories are coming from and seeing which are easier to eliminate. Knowing the calorie content can help you make informed choices guided by your values.

Knowledge is power.

CHAPTER 3

A Model for Understanding Weight Control

The control of our weight is centred in our brain and dictated by our genetic makeup and our environment. As it happens, there are three areas of the brain that are responsible for our food intake and weight regulation. There is a very primitive area of our brain called the hypothalamus, and this structure may be looked at as our appetite centre. It tells us when we are hungry and it tells us when we are satiated, that is when we are full. The hypothalamus does this by regulating our weight around a weight set point. This is analogous to the temperature set point of a thermostat. This setpoint is genetically determined, although it can be modified by environmental influences. The medication I use to help patients lose weight acts on the hypothalamus as it lowers the weight set point in the hypothalamus. Now, this appetite centre of the brain is also referred to as the gatekeeper and the gatekeeper guards against weight loss which it sees as a threat to your survival. So, when this structure detects weight loss it sounds a neurohormonal biological alarm to stimulate our appetite and to seek food to prevent weight loss and to stimulate regain of the lost weight.

So, when you're on medication and your body weight starts dropping, the hypothalamus, the gatekeeper, doesn't get upset and sound the alarm because your weight set point has been lowered by the medication. For folks with weight trouble, it's as though the setpoint is set too high for them.

The second area of the brain that is responsible for food intake is called the mesolimbic system sometimes referred to as the pleasure-reward system. Others have described this area of the brain as the "go-getter" or "hunter" part of the brain, and it gives rise to the wanting or craving of food, and it motivates us to seek food.

To illustrate the mesolimbic system at work, I'd like to give you a personal example. I just finished a lovely meal. I am pleasantly full and I am not hungry but you have just placed a chocolate bar in front of me. Now I'm going to eat that chocolate bar, not because I'm hungry, but because it's pleasurable for me to eat it. Because it tastes good and I enjoy eating it. I might even wrestle you for it. Such is the power of the mesolimbic system. Now, in some folks with weight trouble, it's thought that the "volume" on their mesolimbic system is turned up too high. The good news is that the medication that I use can help you turn down the volume on the mesolimbic system.

It's been really interesting in that patients report to me that they no longer have strong cravings for their particular food. For example, I've had patients tell me that they no longer crave potato chips, and no longer eat them, or that maybe they can have just a few chips and they're done eating them.

I've also had feedback from several patients that their desire for alcohol has become much less. Their habit had been to have three or four beers over the course of an evening, but since the medication, they just don't fancy a beer or maybe they will only have one and then they're done, they're satisfied. The medication helps control the cravings and allows you to follow the nutritionist advice without white-knuckling the day-to-day eating. Wouldn't that be nice?

Now, the third area of the brain that plays an important role in our food intake and weight control is the prefrontal cortex. The prefrontal cortex is the thinking area of our brain and it's referred to as the executive functioning area. Executive functioning includes focussing our attention, predicting the consequences of our actions, impulse control, along with managing emotional reactions and planning for the future.

Now in our model, I want you to picture an important executive sitting behind his desk – but unfortunately for many, the executive is asleep at his desk, although there is a computer sitting on his desk on autopilot mode. So, for many folks with weight trouble, their executive is sleepy and their computer is making automatic decisions for them. This is what is meant by the term mindless eating. Prior to every behaviour, there is a thought, so if we can change the thinking, the premise is that we can change the behaviour. Losing weight is about changing behaviour.

In another section, we will talk more about ways of awakening the sleepy executive and allowing more mindful eating or what I like to call training the brain to think like a thin person. The reality is the conscious brain cannot access or influence our hypothalamus or our mesolimbic system, although as mentioned, the medication I use for my patients can access both of those areas.

The other good news is that our conscious mind can access our prefrontal cortex, so there is an opportunity here for interaction at this level. Such intervention is broadly called cognitive restructuring or changing how you think. This model of changing how you think is utilized in psychology to help patients with depression, anxiety and adult attention deficit hyperactivity disorder. It is a useful intervention that has been validated not only for these psychological-emotional troubles but also as being helpful in weight loss.

CHAPTER 4

Cognitive Restructuring

So today I'm going to discuss cognitive restructuring and how it can be a powerful technique to help you reach your weight loss goals. But what does the term mean? Simply put it means changing the way you think. Changing the way you think is an important treatment approach to helping you lose weight. Now cognitive restructuring was first developed by the well-known American psychiatrist Dr. Aaron Beck who developed the cognitive restructuring technique known as Cognitive Behavioural Therapy or CBT for short. He developed this therapy to help his patients with depression and anxiety disorders, and this technique is now utilized by psychiatrists, psychologists and counsellors the world over. It has been proven to be beneficial for helping the disorders of depression, anxiety and adult attention deficit hyperactivity disorder.

Now, Dr. Aaron Beck has a daughter whose name is Dr. Judith Beck and she is a clinical psychologist who applied the principles of her father's Cognitive Behavioural Therapy to weight management. This proved to be helpful and now Dr. Judith Beck is also a well-known mental health professional who has helped many patients with weight trouble, to lose weight. Dr.

Judith Beck coined the phrase "training the brain to think like a thin person", and this is a useful description of cognitive restructuring as applied to weight management. Cognitive behavioural therapy for weight management teaches the patient to think differently, to help overcome common dietary pitfalls and sabotaging thoughts. It helps to give the patient a sense of confidence and motivation to follow a healthy diet and an active lifestyle for the long term.

Although cognitive behavioural therapy is very beneficial for weight management there is another cognitive restructuring therapy that works even better. It's called acceptance and commitment therapy or simply acceptance-based therapy and this technique was developed by another American psychologist, Dr. Steven Hayes. Acceptance and commitment therapy has also been applied to weight management and its benefit for weight loss has also been validated in clinical studies.

Depending on the study you look at, study subjects had an average weight loss of anywhere from 9% to 14% of their body weight, with cognitive restructuring being the only intervention. When you add acceptance and commitment therapy to our medication program you get a synergistic benefit. So, acceptance and commitment therapy is the cognitive restructuring therapy that I endorse, and it is also the therapy utilized by Lisa Chilvers, the nutritionist who helps me with managing my weight-loss patients.

Acceptance and commitment therapy for weight loss utilizes the concepts of mindful eating and the discovery of values to help guide the direction of eating behaviours. You are guided to accept your reaction and feelings, even if they are negative, and guide you to choose a valued direction and then to take action. An example of this might be the scenario where you were presented with a slice of chocolate cake. You acknowledge that the chocolate cake is very tasty and that you want it. You don't try to suppress this feeling or deny that you want it and that it tastes good; you acknowledge it.

However, you pause, and you reflect on your values: I want to eat healthily so I'll live longer and be there for my grandchildren. So, after reflecting on your values and acknowledging your food desire, you choose to have the tasty mandarin orange instead.

This actually reminds me that I wanted to discuss with you the process of wanting, that is wanting a desired food. Think of wanting as a wave. The wave builds up, crests then falls. This is true of wanting food as well. If we resist the wanting of a desired food, the desire builds up to a crest, and if we continue to resist, it does eventually fall and dissipate. This resistance to wanting takes practice and repetition. While initially being difficult, with time it becomes easier. This is the process of training the brain akin to the physical training of a muscle. Initially, it is difficult, and your muscles are sore, but over time it becomes easier as the muscles adapt and become stronger. Eventually, it becomes relatively effortless and even second nature.

Neural networks for desirable behaviour are strengthened and neural networks for undesirable behaviour over time are weakened. The undesirable behaviour is gradually replaced by the desirable behaviour. For acceptance and commitment therapy to be effective, you have to have a willingness to accept this method. If you have the attitude "Nope, I'm not going to accept any discomfort at all, even for my own good," then obviously this method can't help you lose weight above and beyond the weight loss from the medication alone. Change the dialogue in your head from "if only" to "even if". For example, instead of saying to yourself, "I'd go for a walk if only I wasn't tired" to "I'll go for a walk even if I am tired."

Acceptance and commitment therapy helps you challenge your automatic beliefs and thoughts. Acceptance and commitment therapy helps you identify your values and you can use your decision-making as a vote in favour of your treasured values. Remember: a goal is a destination that once reached, motivation dissipates, whereas a value is the direction that you want to move towards, and that serves you for the rest of your life.

Contact Lisa Chilvers for support in this area and collaborate with her. You can contact her through her website lisachilvers.ca. Lisa will assist you in this mindfulness approach and assist you in developing the skills of resilience and restraint, along with helping you to develop a healthy eating lifestyle. As mentioned previously, her methodology has a little twist on acceptance and commitment therapy that she calls The Loving Kindness Method. Patients love it – and what's more, it works.

CHAPTER 5

Modulators of Weight Regulation

There are a number of modulators of appetite and weight regulation that I have to be mindful about when seeing a patient. These modulators need to be identified and addressed as an aid to assist the patient in trying to lose weight. I think many of us have experienced emotional eating and can relate to what I'm about to discuss. For some folks, eating isn't just about satisfying physical hunger.

At times of stress, we may turn to food to comfort us. There's a term for such food: comfort food, which often tends to be high-calorie, high-carbohydrate sweet foods. You might be eating for comfort if you're bored or lonely. As infants, when we cried, one of the first things our mothers would do is feed us to try and get us to stop crying and to comfort us this way. We have been conditioned from an early age to use food to comfort ourselves. The more extreme example of this is the patient with binge-eating disorder who overstuffs themselves with food in an effort to reduce their emotional distress. Unfortunately, overeating can lead to feelings of self-loathing and disgust which can further lower the patient's spirits, driving them to eat even more for comfort in a vicious cycle.

Some folks when they're depressed have a reduced appetite and actually lose weight, and some folks with anxiety have reduced appetite and also lose weight. However, many folks who suffer from depression and suffer from chronic anxiety have an increase in their food intake and experience weight gain. Clearly, to help the patient lose weight, the patient's depression and anxiety disorder or stressful situation needs to be addressed and appropriately treated.

When patients are significantly depressed, they lose interest, they lose motivation and this greatly interferes with the successful management of weight loss. I usually advise treatment for depression first, and once the depression is in remission, I then start medical weight loss management. If you eat to reward yourself, if you eat to make yourself feel better temporarily, if you eat because you're bored, if you feel guilty after you eat, you likely are experiencing emotional eating. Emotional eating behaviours can be helped by the acceptance and commitment therapy that I was discussing in the previous session.

Sleep deprivation: I see so many patients with weight trouble who are very poor sleepers. Unfortunately, poor sleep can be an important cause of weight gain. Clearly, poor sleep doesn't cause weight gain in everybody, but it is a major risk factor for weight gain. When you sleep poorly your body makes more of the hunger hormone called ghrelin and it makes less of the satiety hormone called leptin. So, when you are not getting a good night's rest, your body makes you more hungry and less easy to satisfy. A good number of my more severely obese patients get less than four hours sleep a night total, and they have been like that for years. This is their normal. If you are sleeping poorly, please see your doctor for management of your sleep disorder as the treatment of your insomnia is critical to the success of your weight management. This discussion reminds me of that old adage: "Work eight hours, play eight hours and rest eight hours". The adage might be old, but it is still a wise regimen to live by today.

It is thought that there are chemicals in our environment that get into our food chain that disrupt the normal hormonal regulation of our appetite. It is theorized that these chemicals are an important contribution to the weight gain seen in our society. The chemicals are collectively referred to as endocrine-disrupting chemicals and they include pesticides, phthalates, PCBs, and bisphenols. These synthetic chemicals disrupt the normal function and production of hormones that are involved in weight regulation, and this can contribute to our obesity.
An example here is the use of bisphenol A that is used as a coating that lines cans and plastic food and plastic beverage containers. This is why beverage containers should be glass or metal and not plastic and why you should store food in glass rather than plastic containers.

Now for many of you, a biggie that is modulating your appetite and weight control is medication. Some medications can have a very detrimental effect on your weight and hence your weight-loss efforts.

Many of you may be on anti-depressant therapy and on it for a very good reason, so I'm not advocating that you stop. So many antidepressant medications are weight-promoting, while others are not, or are less likely to cause weight gain. If you are on antidepressant medication, the thing to do is to have a conversation with your prescribing doctor and see if your medication might be switched if you happen to be on a weight-promoting antidepressant.

The antidepressants that I believe tend to promote weight gain in some patients are the SSRI medications like paroxetine, citalopram and escitalopram. The SNRI medications like duloxetine and venlafaxine and the tricyclic antidepressants like amitriptyline and imipramine are also weight-promoting. The SNRIs tend to be less troublesome than the SSRIs with respect to weight promotion. The novel antidepressant mirtazapine is notorious for weight gain and even trazodone can cause modest weight gain. Trazodone is often used as a sleep aid rather than as a pure antidepressant because it has quite strong sedative side effects that are taken advantage of to help the patient sleep. The antidepressant bupropion does not cause weight gain and may contribute to very modest weight loss. Unfortunately, I haven't found bupropion very helpful as an anti-depressant but have used it as an augmenting agent to augment the benefit of the primary antidepressant.

The newer antidepressants like vortioxetine and levomilnacipran are reported to not be associated with weight gain.

When it comes to treating depression there are a number of factors to consider, so any medication changes should be done in consultation with your family doctor or your psychiatrist. Do not stop your antidepressant. Discuss the issues with your doctor. Quite often antidepressants do not put the patient into full remission and so the doctor will often prescribe a so-called atypical antipsychotic medication to augment the beneficial effects of the primary antidepressant. In this case, we then call the medications augmenting agents.

Unfortunately, most atypical antipsychotics when added to an SSRI or an SNRI will cause a very significant weight gain. These atypical antipsychotics can be extremely helpful in assisting the patient get into full remission from the depression, so again, please do not stop if you happen to be taking one of the weight-promoting augmenting medications. Please discuss with your doctor. Common weight-promoting antipsychotics include quetiapine, risperidone, aripiprazole and olanzapine. All of the atypical antipsychotic medications tend to promote weight gain with the exception of ziprasidone.

Atypical antipsychotic medications are often used by themselves when they are used to treat the major mental illnesses of schizophrenia and manic-depressive disorder. In this situation, they too can be weight-promoting. If you suffer from one of these disorders, you must not stop taking your medication as it is essential for your well-being. Please instead discuss the issue with your psychiatrist.

I do wish to point out that I have successfully treated patients with weight-loss medication in spite of them taking weight-promoting medication including the taking of atypical antipsychotics. So, it is not essential that the atypical antipsychotic medications be stopped in order to get successful weight loss. The atypical antipsychotic medication brexpiprazole is also used as an adjunct to antidepressant treatment, and it's interesting to see that treatment with this medication tends to cause weight gain in those who were initially underweight or normal weight whereas those who were already overweight or obese didn't gain any further weight.

So, we have implicated the antidepressants. We have implicated the antipsychotics. The next anti-medication class that is weight-promoting are the antihistamines. All antihistamines can promote weight gain except fexofenadine, trade name Allegra® as it does not cross the blood-brain barrier to exert an appetite-stimulating effect in our brain. So, if you suffer from hay fever, you do want to try to get the most out of allergy nose spray and allergy eye drops and avoidance of the offending allergen and rely less on antihistamines. If you do need to use an antihistamine, then Allegra would be a weight-friendly choice.

Hyposensitization therapy, supervised by an allergist, is also a good alternative treatment if your allergies are severe.

There are several anticonvulsant medications that seem to also promote weight gain, but if you suffer from epilepsy it is essential that you remain on the medication. However, many patients are prescribed anticonvulsant medications for other reasons like for the treatment of fibromyalgia, neuropathic pain syndromes like sciatica and for chronic headache syndromes. The medications gabapentin and pregabalin are examples of such medication that are used for these pain syndromes that are weight-promoting.

There are alternative medications that could be considered to treat these pain syndromes that are not weight-promoting. You should discuss the issue with your doctor to see if an alternative can be used. In some cases, there is no alternative that is as effective. Lamotrigine is an anticonvulsant that is not thought to cause weight gain and it is also used as a mood stabilizer in those suffering from bipolar disorder.

We are now going to discuss anti-diabetic medications. Some anti-diabetic medications do promote weight gain. Many folks with type two diabetes are either overweight or obese and the doctor is routinely telling such patients that losing weight will help their diabetes. The doctor might then turn around and prescribe weight-promoting anti-diabetic medication. The sulphonylurea class of medications like gliclazide and glyburide promote weight gain. The TZD medications pioglitazone and rosiglitazone also promote weight gain. Insulin promotes weight gain. Do not stop your diabetic medications. Instead, have a discussion with your diabetes doctor.

It might be appropriate to switch your medication to an anti-diabetic medication that can promote weight loss or that is at least weight neutral. The anti-diabetic medication class known as the SGLT2 inhibitors like canagliflozin, dapagliflozin and empagliflozin are all modest weight-losing diabetic medications. They do not help the non-diabetic patient to lose weight.

The diabetic medication class referred to as the GLP1 agonists can cause significant weight loss in both the diabetic and the non-diabetic patient. Medications in this class include Victoza®, Saxenda®, Trulicity®, Ozempic®, Adlyxin® and Bydureon®.

The beta-blocker class of medication can also promote weight gain. This class of medication is used in the treatment of high blood pressure, heart disease and sometimes for migraine headache prophylaxis. Do NOT stop your beta-blocker. Doing so can be dangerous. Instead, have a discussion with your doctor and see if any medication can be substituted and the beta-blocker tapered off.

If you're taking a beta-blocker for heart disease you probably cannot come off this medication. Examples of this class of medication include propranolol, atenolol, bisoprolol, metoprolol and others.

The steroid hormones prednisone and dexamethasone are also powerful promoters of weight gain, but if you're on one of these medications you have a very good medical justification for being on them. Follow your doctor's directions and advice. This is not an exhaustive list of medications that promote weight gain, but it covers the main offenders.

I'd like to emphasize by way of repeating myself: do not stop any weight-promoting medication yourself. Do discuss with your doctor to see if there are alternative treatments for your condition that may not demand a weight-promoting medication. Your doctor is the best person to advise you if any changes can be safely made because they understand your particular medical situ

CHAPTER 6

Weight Loss Medication

When it comes to weight loss, I find that most people do much better with the aid of medication for weight management. In Canada, there are only three medications officially approved for weight management. They are:

- Orlistat, trade name Xenical®

- combination of bupropion and naltrexone, trade name Contrave®, and

- liraglutide, trade name Saxenda®.

In other countries, there may be other options. Although I don't have experience with those other options, I sincerely doubt that they work as well as the medication I now most commonly use. The medication I use is not an approved medication for use as a weight-loss drug at the present moment any place in the world. This is an important consideration in that what I am doing hasn't been sanctioned by any health authority at the present time.

The medication is however approved as a treatment for type 2 diabetes mellitus. The medication I most commonly use and find the most effective is called semaglutide, which is sold under the trade name Ozempic®. Semaglutide is approved by various health authorities for the management of type 2 diabetes. Semaglutide is under development and investigation for weight management and for the treatment of fatty liver disease but is not yet approved to treat these conditions.

I felt comfortable using the medication semaglutide for weight loss after the Phase 2 dose-finding study was published in the British medical journal, The Lancet. The efficacy data and the safety data from that study suggested to me that it was a more potent medication than Saxenda and that the safety profile and side-effect profile was virtually the same as Saxenda. Saxenda was the medication I had most commonly used in weight management for my patients. I was also already experienced in using semaglutide for the management of my patients with type 2 diabetes.

At the time of this writing, the Phase 3 studies for semaglutide as a weight-loss drug are concluding, and the Step 4 study results have recently been released. Results of this Phase 3 study further reassures me on the safety and efficacy of semaglutide as a weight-loss medication.

In my experience of using semaglutide as an anti-diabetic medication, I was very impressed by how powerful a drug this was in helping correct my diabetic patients' blood sugars and also seeing significant associated weight loss in these diabetic patients. Now the maximum dose of Ozempic® used to treat type two diabetes is 1 mg weekly; yes – only once a week dosing. For weight loss though, the maximum dose I use is 2.5 mg weekly, a dose significantly higher than what is approved for the treatment of diabetes. Furthermore, the dose used in the Step 4 study was 2.4 mg weekly and the average weight loss in that study was 17%. Of course, this is an average weight loss. Some patients did better, and some patients did not do as well.

My patients who receive semaglutide and follow my exercise prescription and see Lisa Chilvers for nutritional counselling and acceptance and commitment therapy counselling, are seeing weight loss in the 26% to 28% range after about 9 to 12 months of therapy. The occasional patient has lost 30% of their weight. This degree of weight loss is unprecedented in my weight loss practice.

Bariatric surgery I believe is the only other intervention that can result in more weight loss than this program that I am currently following.

- Gastric sleeve surgery results in about a 20% to 30% weight loss.

- Roux-en-Y gastric bypass surgery generally results in a 25% to 35% weight loss.

And

- Biliopancreatic diversion with duodenal switch surgery results in a 30% to 40% weight loss.

Bariatric surgery clearly gives rise to impressive results, but unfortunately, this comes with an increased risk. There is the possibility of surgical complications with every surgical procedure and for bariatric surgery, one of those complications can be death.

The operative mortality risk (meaning death within 30 days of surgery) is:

- 1/1000 for gastric sleeve surgery

- 5/1000 for Roux-en-Y gastric bypass surgery, and

- 11/1000 for Biliopancreatic diversion with duodenal switch surgery.

If you decide to have surgery, make sure you have a very experienced surgeon as the more experienced the surgeon, the less the risk.

The other issue with surgery is weight regain. This is more likely with gastric sleeve surgery, somewhat likely with Roux-en-Y gastric bypass surgery and less likely with the biliopancreatic diversion with duodenal switch surgery.

In one study, 59% of patients who underwent Roux-en-Y gastric bypass surgery regained at least 20% of the weight lost. Certainly, I've seen patients present at the highest weight in their life, five years or more following Roux-en-Y gastric bypass surgery.

With more robust medication available and improved psychological therapy and support, non-operative medical intervention is becoming a viable option for many who suffer from obesity.

Now let's get back to talking about the medication semaglutide. When I prescribe this medication, I am prescribing it "off label". Both the indication and the dose are off label. This means that semaglutide is not approved for weight management and the dose is not approved for any indication by Health Canada. Doctors are allowed to prescribe medication "off label" as long as they inform the patient that it is off label, and I can tell you that physicians very often prescribe medications off label presumably when they believe that the benefit outweighs the risk in each individual patient's case.

Now, I'm licensed to practice medicine only in the province of Ontario, Canada, so if you live outside of Ontario I cannot prescribe to you, so you will need to see your own doctor to get a prescription. It's possible that your own doctor may not feel comfortable prescribing semaglutide off label to you. If this is the

case, I'd suggest using Saxenda® instead which would be on label for weight management, as long as your body mass index is 30 or greater, or 27 or greater in the presence of at least one weight-related morbidity – for example, high blood pressure, type 2 diabetes or high cholesterol.
The patient should also have failed at least one previous weight-management intervention, according to the label.

Liraglutide, trade name Saxenda®, was my favourite weight-loss medication before I switched to semaglutide, trade name Ozempic®. Both medications are injectable using a pen device called a FlexTouch® pen and the needles that I prescribe for this pen are called NovoFine Plus® Needles. The pen technology and the NovoFine Plus® needles are brilliant.

When you use this pen device, it literally does not hurt to self-inject. Nobody seems to believe me when I tell them, but it's true. It does not hurt. Saxenda is injected every day and Ozempic® is injected once a week. The two medications have a lot in common. They belong to the same class of medications called GLP1 receptor agonists. This means that they stimulate the GLP1 receptors located in the pancreas and the brain.

The clever thing about this medication is that if your sugar level is normal, it doesn't act on the pancreas. This way, non-diabetic patients don't have to worry that the sugar will go too low. How clever is that? How cool is that? Ozempic® appears to be more robust than Saxenda® in stimulating these GLP1 receptors and the appetite centres in the brain that results in less hunger, quicker satiety and less craving.

Let's now talk about the side effects of the medication. Saxenda® and Ozempic® are very similar, with the main side effects being nausea, vomiting, constipation and diarrhea. To mitigate the side effects we start both medications at a low dose and gradually titrate the dose up, as long as the patient is tolerating them.

Because there is no label for titrating Ozempic® to 2.5 mg, I decided to use the following regimen, which seems to work quite well in that it is well tolerated by the majority of patients. Some patients may experience mild nausea that's transient and manageable when the medication is used this way. For Ozempic®:

- I start with the dose of 0.25 mg once a week for a month

- then I titrate the dose up to 0.5 mg weekly for a month

- and then I increase it to 1 mg weekly for a month

- then 1.5 mg weekly for a month

- then 2 mg weekly for a month

- and then, finally, after 5 months, 2.5 mg weekly as the long-term maintenance dose.

In the Phase 3 study called the Step 4 study, the dose of semaglutide was 2.4 mg weekly as the long-term maintenance dose. I chose the 2.5 mg dose for simplicity in guiding patients. The FlexTouch® pens are not currently designed to give 2.5 mg or 2.4 mg as a single dose, because I am using the pens off label.

The pens come in 2 different sizes. There is the 2mg pen that can administer 0.25 mg or 0.5mg dose and then there is the 4mg pen that is designed to only administer the 1mg dose.
To administer 2.5 mg of Ozempic® I have the patient administer two 1mg doses from the 4 mg pen and one 0.5mg dose from the 2mg pen to make a total of 2.5mg.

Alternatively, the patient uses the 4mg pen to administer two doses of 1 mg and then using the same pen dials up 35 clicks of the pen which approximates 0.5mg and then administers that. This latter technique is more prone to dosing error, but it turns out that this technique is cheaper and if you're a cash-paying patient, you really appreciate that.

If this is all too confusing, your doctor or pharmacist should be able to help guide you to give the correct dose. As you are titrating the dose, do not increase the dose even if scheduled, if you are only just tolerating the current dose. Wait until you feel well before increasing the dose higher. Also, if you are not tolerating a certain dose, step down to the next lower level that you did tolerate, and after a few weeks, try raising the dose again.

The occasional patient will use Gravo®l to help relieve any nausea, and some patients need to use a laxative like RestoraLax® to help combat constipation if that becomes an issue.

Okay, but what about the safety of the medications Saxenda® and Ozempic® you ask? The safety concerns of Saxenda® and Ozempic® are the same. In rat and mice studies, both medications do show an association between drug exposure and the development of thyroid cancer. That, of course, sounds very concerning, but fortunately, there is no evidence whatsoever that these medications cause or can cause thyroid cancer in humans. Indeed, neither Health Canada nor the FDA would have approved the use of these medications if they suspected that they could cause cancer in humans. (If you were a rodent, then there would definitely be a concern).

What is a real safety concern is the increased risk of developing gallstones and symptomatic gallbladder disease and acute pancreatitis. Folks who lose a significant amount of weight for any reason are at an increased risk of developing gallstones in the gallbladder. This can then trigger gallbladder attacks severe enough to warrant surgical removal of the gallbladder. Very occasionally a gallstone will escape the gallbladder and block the pancreatic duct and trigger acute pancreatitis which is a potentially life-threatening illness. Fortunately, none of my weight-loss patients have developed pancreatitis and I believe it is a very uncommon complication of therapy.

Now that covers the relevant safety concerns, so let's now talk about other benefits of these medications. Both medications have been proven in medical studies to reduce the risk of heart attack, stroke, and death in the diabetic population. At the time of this writing, there is no completed study proving the cardiovascular benefit of these medications in the obese non-diabetic population. Since obese patients are at increased cardiovascular risk, it is likely that cardiovascular risk reduction is also a benefit from these medications in the non-diabetic population as well. These medications have been proven to reduce the risk of developing diabetes and pre-diabetes.

All in all, and on balance, pretty good stuff. So who should not be taking these medications? Well,

- if you are pregnant or nursing, you should not be taking any GLP1 agonist, including Saxenda® and Ozempic®.

- If you have a personal or family history of medullary thyroid cancer, then you should not be taking any GLP1 agonist.

- If you have a personal or family history of multiple endocrine neoplasia syndrome type 2, then you should not take these medications.

- If you are under the age of 18 then this medication is not for you, as it has not been tested in your age group.

Patients often ask me how long they need to be taking the medication for. Please understand that being overweight is a chronic medical condition, and you require lifelong treatment. Will you remain on Ozempic® for the rest of your life? No, as there are even more powerful medications in the pipeline that are coming that will help you lose even more weight if needed. You do require lifelong treatment if you suffer from the medical condition of obesity.

This is an exciting time to be alive! It's an exciting time for weight loss, as better medication is coming to the marketplace in the not-too-distant future. Current treatment works very well, and we will have even better tools within the next few years.

I'd like to finish by summarizing some key concepts about weight management that you should keep in mind.

1) Many folks are not able to achieve the so-called ideal weight, so please focus instead on looking for your personal best weight that can be achieved with the best medication available and best cognitive restructuring therapy available while following the healthiest lifestyle that you can still enjoy.

2) A typical diet is the smallest number of calories and the greatest amount of exercise that a person can endure, while a healthy lifestyle is the smallest number of calories and the greatest amount of activity that you can enjoy. Remember, if you do not enjoy your lifestyle, you will not be able to maintain it in the long term, and this is why diets almost always fail. A normal person – and you are a normal person – cannot tolerate a diet for long if they don't enjoy it.

3) The use of medication to help you lose weight and maintain that loss is not an admission of personal failure, but a recognition that being overweight is a real medical condition that can benefit from proper medical treatment.

4) If you have failed to lose weight and keep it off in the past, do not consider that you are a personal failure, that you are weak-willed or somehow inferior. Consider that you are human, and you simply never received the proper treatment that included the best medication available and the best cognitive restructuring therapy available.

If you live in Ontario and if you wish to see me for a weight-management consultation, then I suggest that you ask your family doctor to refer you to me at Fax: 226-319-134. If you wish to provide feedback to me which I welcome, then please contact me through my website triadweightlossclinic.com. If patients anywhere in the world wish to see Lisa Chilvers (virtually) for nutritional counselling, combined with cognitive restructuring therapy that she calls The Loving Kindness Method, then contact her by visiting her website at lisachilvers.ca

If you enjoyed this book on modern medical weight management and find it useful or educational, then please share the book with your family, friends and neighbours, who you think may be interested in reading

Acknowledgement

I'd like to give credit to the following leading experts in medical weight loss in Canada.:

- Dr. David Macklin of the Medcan Weight Management Program in Toronto
- Dr. Arya Sharma, Professor of Medicine at the University of Alberta, and the founder of Obesity Canada
- Dr. Michael Vallis, Clinical Psychologist and Associate Professor at Dalhousie University, and
- Dr. Yoni Freedhoff, Professor of Family Medicine at the University of Ottawa.

They are amongst the leading experts in medical weight loss in Canada. I appreciate all their teachings. They have helped me understand modern medical weight loss management and their thinking has helped guide my approach to medical weight management.

Special thanks to my daughter Lisa Chilvers R.H.N. for her feedback, guidance and support in the writing of this book.
 Lastly, I'd like to thank my wife Maria Chilvers whose encouragement, love and support helps me in everything I do.

About the Author

Dr. Martyn Chilvers retired from family practice in 2015 after 32 years to become the medical director of the Triad Weight Loss Clinic located in Sarnia, Ontario, Canada. He has helped hundreds of patients successfully lose weight and keep it off. In 2018 he received the 'Patient's Choice Award' as an acknowledgement of his excellence in patient care. He lives in Sarnia with his wife Maria.

www.ingramcontent.com/pod-product-compliance
Lightning Source LLC
Chambersburg PA
CBHW051418250726
48655CB00003B/1112